THE COMPLETE PLANT-BASED DIET COOKBOOK

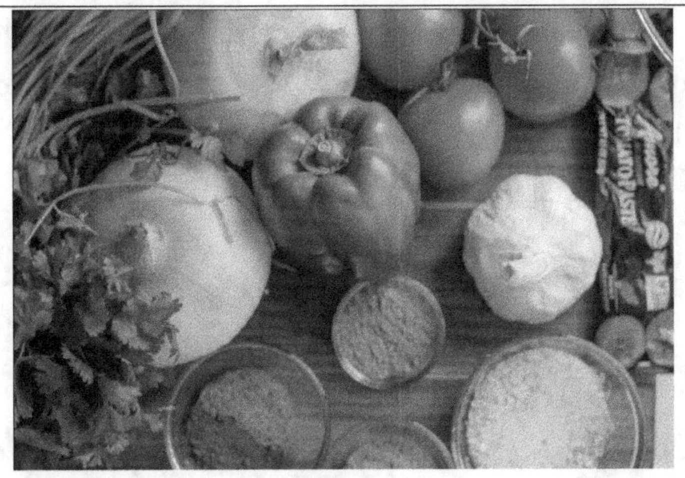

Vegan and Vegetarian Recipe for a Healthy Lifestyle

Anna Moss

Copyright © 2023 by Anna Moss

All rights reserved

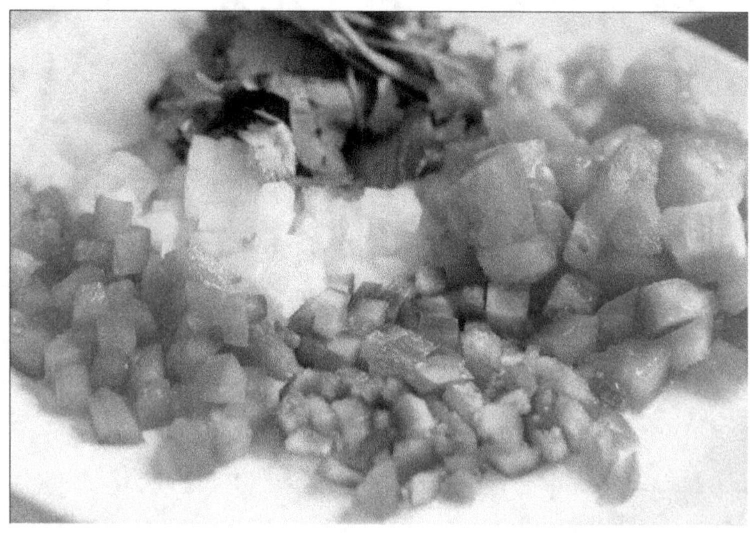

Table of Contents

INTRODUCTION

Once upon a time, there was a young woman named Liana who had been struggling with her health for many years. She had tried countless diets and remedies, but nothing seemed to work. She was feeling desperate and lost, until one day she stumbled across Anna Moss plant-based diet cookbook while browsing the internet.

The cookbook promised to provide Liana with all the necessary recipes and information to transform her health and lifestyle. She was intrigued, and so she purchased the book and began to explore its pages.

What Liana found was a world of deliciousness that she never knew existed. She discovered recipes for things like Coconut curry noodle bowl, Marinated Tofu, Baked Sweet Potato & Black Bean Burrito. She was amazed at the variety of flavors and textures that she could create from such simple ingredients.

She also found information about the health benefits of a plant-based diet, including weight loss, reduced inflammation, and improved energy levels. She was inspired to make some real, lasting changes to her lifestyle.

Within a few weeks, Liana had completely transformed her diet. She was eating more fruits and vegetables than ever before, and she had even started growing her own herbs and vegetables in her garden. She felt healthier and happier than she ever had before.

Anna Moss plant-based diet cookbook had been a real game-changer for Liana. She had found a way to improve her health and wellbeing, and she was grateful for the guidance it had provided. She was now living a healthier, happier life.

Welcome to Plant-Based Diet Cookbook! This cookbook is designed to help you make delicious, healthy, and nutritious plant-based meals that are easy to prepare.

This cookbook includes a variety of vegan, vegetarian, and flexitarian recipes that are suitable for all skill levels. Whether you're completely new to plant-based cooking or have some experience, you'll find something to enjoy here.

The recipes in this cookbook are made with wholesome, real-food ingredients that are mostly or entirely plant-based. This means all the recipes are free from animal products, including eggs, dairy, and honey.

We've divided the cookbook into sections to make it easier to find the recipes you're looking for. You'll find breakfast recipes, lunch recipes, dinner recipes, snacks, sides, and desserts.

We've also included helpful tips and tricks throughout the cookbook to help make preparing your meals easier. We hope you find this cookbook helpful and that you discover some delicious new meals to add to your repertoire.

Enjoy!

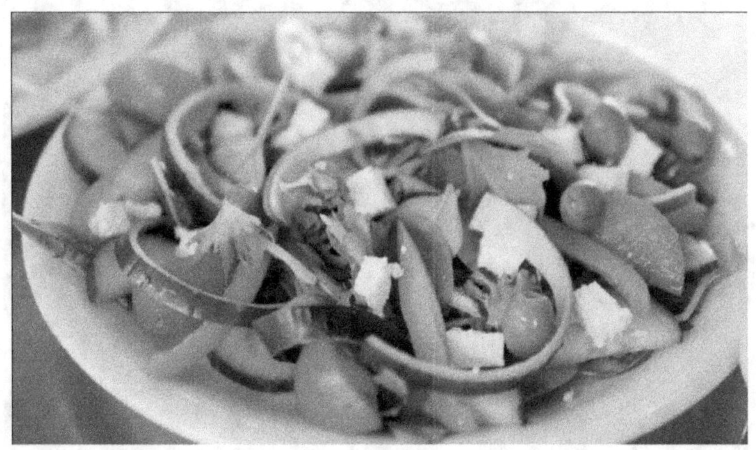

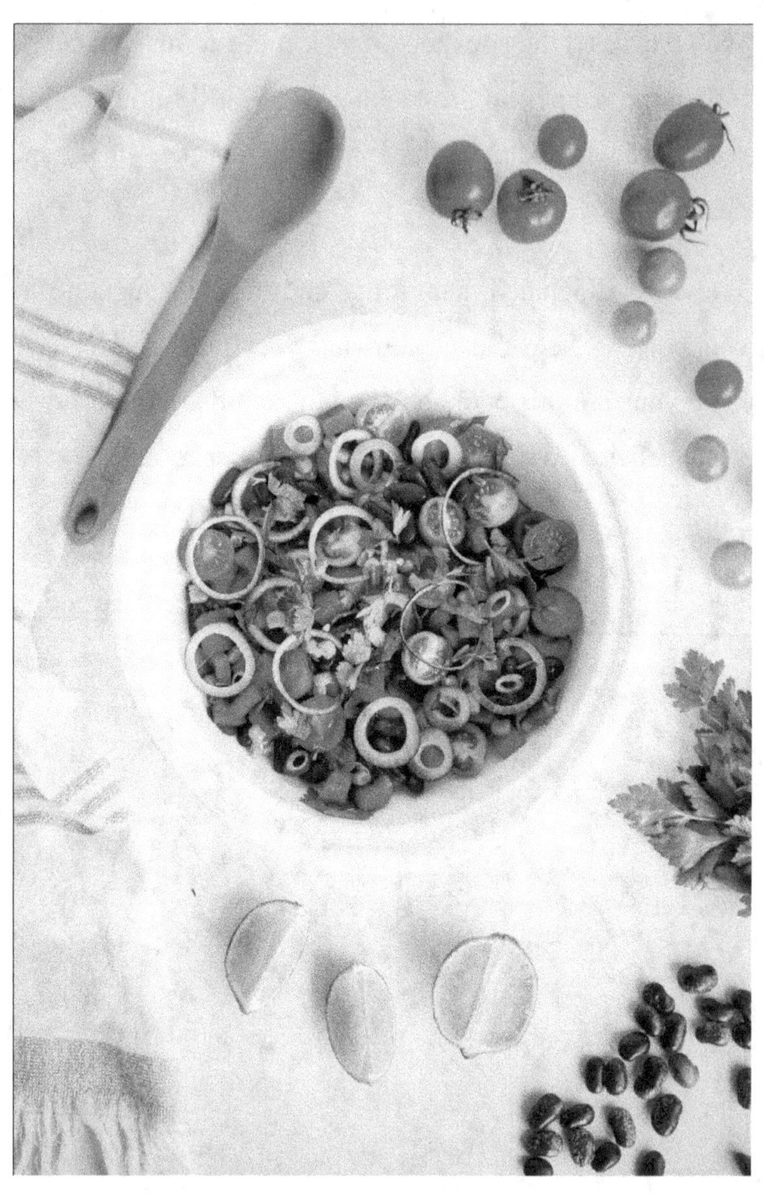

CHAPTER 1

Getting started with plant-based eating

Plant-based eating is a way of eating that focuses on consuming whole, unprocessed plants. This type of diet is becoming increasingly popular due to its health benefits, environmental sustainability, and ethical considerations.

If you are looking to get started with a plant-based diet, here are some tips to help you make the transition.

1. Start slow: Don't try to change your entire diet overnight. Start by introducing more plant-based foods into your routine and slowly reduce your consumption of animal products. You can also start by reducing the amount of meat you eat in one meal and replacing it with plant-based proteins such as beans, lentils, tofu, and tempeh.

2. Focus on whole foods: Plant-based eating focuses on whole, unprocessed foods. Ditch processed foods, refined sugars, and unhealthy fats and focus on eating whole grains, vegetables, fruits, nuts, and legumes.

3. Experiment with new recipes: Cooking plant-based meals doesn't have to be boring or intimidating. Try experimenting with different herbs and spices to create different flavors.

4. Don't be afraid to supplement: If you are worried about missing out on certain nutrients, consider supplementing your diet with vitamins and minerals. Talk to your doctor or a nutritionist to figure out what supplements you may need.

5. Make it enjoyable: Eating a plant-based diet should be enjoyable. Don't feel like you have to deprive yourself of treats or snacks.

There are plenty of plant-based snacks and desserts that are just as delicious as their animal-based counterparts. By following these tips, you can make the transition to a plant-based diet easier and more enjoyable. With a little bit of effort, you can start to reap the health, environmental, and ethical benefits of eating plant-based.

CHAPTER 2

The science behind a whole food plant based diet

Diets focused on whole, unprocessed plant foods, such as fruits, vegetables, whole grains, legumes, nuts, and seeds, are known as whole-food plant-based diets. These foods are packed with vitamins, minerals, antioxidants, and other beneficial compounds that are key to maintaining good health. Studies have shown that whole food plant-based diets can help prevent and even reverse chronic diseases such as heart disease, type 2 diabetes, and obesity.

The science behind a whole food plant-based diet lies in its ability to provide essential nutrients while keeping calorie intake low. When compared to the average American diet, which is high in processed meats, refined carbohydrates, and unhealthy fats, a whole food plant-based diet is much lower in calories, saturated fat, and cholesterol.

Additionally, whole food plant-based diets are rich in fiber, which helps to reduce cholesterol levels, stabilize blood sugar, and improve digestion.

Other research has found that plant-based diets are beneficial for reducing inflammation, which is linked to many chronic diseases. This is because plant-based diets are rich in antioxidants, which help to reduce oxidative stress and repair damage caused by free radicals. Additionally, plant-based diets are rich in phytochemicals, which have anti-inflammatory effects and can help reduce inflammation-related diseases.

In conclusion, a whole food plant-based diet is a nutritious and health-promoting way of eating. It is associated with a reduced risk of chronic disease, improved digestion, and a reduction in inflammation. Furthermore, it is a diet that is suitable for people of all ages and lifestyles.

How a whole food plant based can significantly boost your health

A whole-foods plant-based diet may dramatically improve your health by giving your body the essential nutrients it needs to perform at its best. Eat full; unprocessed plant-based foods that are high in fiber, vitamins, minerals, antioxidants, and other nutrients are the main focus of this sort of diet.

You may lower your chance of developing chronic illnesses like heart disease, diabetes, and cancer by eating meals that provide your body with vital nutrients. A whole food plant-based diet has also been related to weight loss, improved digestion, and better mental health.

Diets focused on whole foods and plants are considered to be nutrient-dense, meaning they give your body the vitamins and minerals it needs to flourish. A variety of fruits, vegetables, nuts, seeds, legumes, and whole grains should be consumed as part of this diet. These foods are bursting with fiber, vitamins, minerals, antioxidants, and other nutrients that can strengthen your immune system and reduce inflammation. By supplying your body with vital vitamins and minerals, eating these nutrient-dense foods can help lower your chance of developing chronic illnesses.

Additionally, a whole-foods plant-based diet can help your mental health. This kind of diet has a lot of fiber, which can help you feel fuller for longer and reduce your cravings for bad foods. Eating more plant-based meals with high fiber content will also make you feel satisfied for longer, which can result in more stable blood sugar levels, an uplifted mood, and less worry.

Key principle of a plant based diets

The key principle of a plant-based diet is to base the majority of one's food intake on whole, unrefined, and minimally processed plant foods. This means avoiding or minimizing processed and refined foods, including white flour, white sugar, and processed oils. Eating plant-based foods can provide the body with all of the essential vitamins, minerals, and proteins needed for good health.

The key principle of a plant-based diet is to eat a variety of plant-based foods to ensure that the body is getting a wide range of nutrients. This means consuming a variety of whole grains, legumes, nuts, seeds, fruits, and vegetables. Eating a variety of plant-based foods can also help to reduce the risk of developing certain chronic health conditions, such as heart disease, diabetes, and obesity.

In addition to eating a variety of plant-based foods, it is also important to limit consumption of processed and refined foods, as well as animal-based foods. Eating a diet that is low in animal-based foods and high in plant-based foods can help to reduce the risk of developing certain chronic diseases. Additionally, eating plant-based foods can help to reduce the environmental impact of food production and consumption.

Benefits of a Plant Based Diets

A plant-based diet is a way of eating that prioritizes plant-based foods including fruits, vegetables, grains, legumes, seeds, and nuts while reducing or completely excluding animal products like meat, dairy, and eggs.

Some of the benefits of plant-based diets are associated with numerous health benefits, which include:

1. Improved Heart Health: Plant-based diets are naturally rich in heart-healthy vitamins, minerals, and fiber. Studies have shown that these diets can reduce risk factors for heart disease, including high cholesterol, high blood pressure, and obesity.

2. Reduced Risk of Certain Cancers: Eating a plant-based diet may also reduce the risk of developing certain types of cancers. A diet rich in fruits and vegetables is associated with a lower risk of colorectal and stomach cancers.

3. Weight Loss: Plant-based diets are naturally low in calories and are rich in fiber, which can help you feel full for longer and reduce cravings for unhealthy snacks.

Eating a plant-based diet can also help you maintain a healthy weight, and may even result in weight loss.

4. Improved Digestive Health: Eating a plant-based diet is naturally high in fiber, which helps to promote regular bowel movements and reduce the risk of digestive problems such as constipation, diverticulosis, and hemorrhoids.

5. Reduced Risk of Diabetes: Eating a plant-based diet can help reduce the risk of developing type 2 diabetes. Studies have found that plant-based diets are associated with lower levels of blood sugar and improved insulin sensitivity.

6. Reduced Risk of Kidney Disease: Eating a plant-based diet is associated with a reduced risk of developing kidney disease. Plant-based diets are naturally low in sodium and fat, which can help reduce the strain on the kidneys.

7. Improved Mental Health: Eating a plant-based diet has been associated with improved mood and mental clarity. Plant-based diets are naturally high in vitamins and minerals, which can help improve mental health and reduce anxiety and depression.

8. Environmentally Friendly: Eating a plant-based diet is also better for the environment. Plant-based diets require fewer resources, such as water and land, to produce. They also produce fewer greenhouse gas emissions, which can help reduce global warming.

Finally, many people find that plant-based diets can be more enjoyable than diets that include animal products. Plant-based diets offer a variety of flavors, textures, and colors, which can make meals more interesting and enjoyable. Additionally, plant-based diets offer a variety of nutritious and tasty options, which can make it easier to stick to the diet over the long-term.

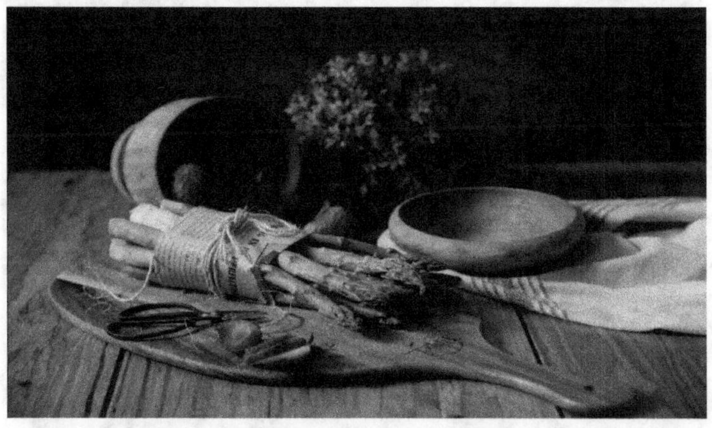

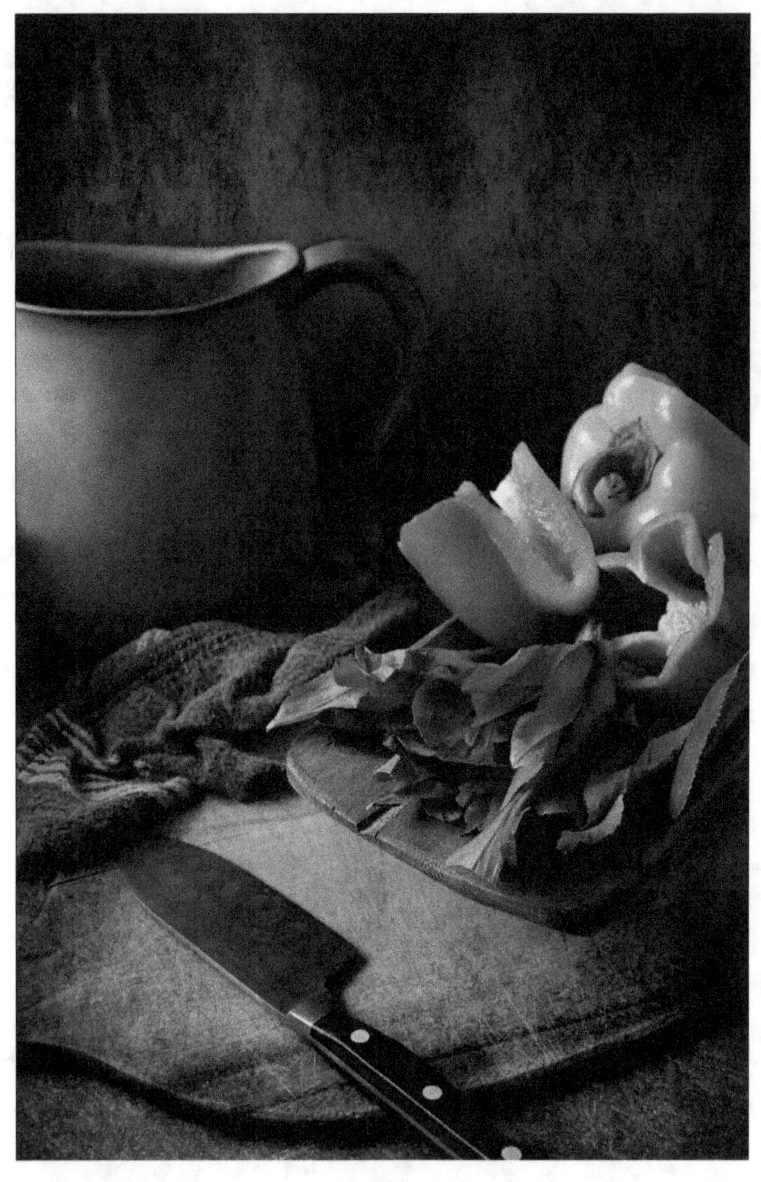

CHAPTER 3

Shopping for Plant-Based Foods

Shopping for plant-based foods can be a great way to improve your health and the environment. Plant-based diets are packed with vitamins, minerals, and other important nutrients, and they are good for your heart and can help reduce your risk of chronic diseases. Plus, they are typically lower in calories than diets that include animal products, making them great for weight management and disease prevention.

When shopping for plant-based foods, you'll want to focus on fresh produce like fruits, vegetables, legumes, nuts, and seeds. These are considered the staples of a plant-based diet and should form the basis of your meals. Be sure to choose a variety of different colored fruits and vegetables, as this will help ensure you're getting a wide range of different vitamins and minerals. If you don't have access to fresh produce, frozen and canned varieties are also good options.

You can also find plant-based proteins, such as tofu, tempeh, lentils, and chickpeas.

These can be used to create delicious plant-based meals that are higher in protein than meals made with just vegetables and grains.

Things to consider when shopping for plant-based items

1. Research different plant-based foods items. Before you shop for plant-based foods, it is important to research the different items and brands available. Read labels carefully to ensure the products contain 100% plant-based ingredients and are free of animal products.

2. Make a list of the items you want to buy. Making a list before you go to the store is a great way to ensure you get everything you need and don't forget any items.

3. Check for coupons and discounts. Many stores offer coupons and discounts for plant-based foods. Look for these before you shop so you can save money.

4. Look for organic or non-GMO products. If you are looking for the healthiest plant-based options, look for organic or non-GMO labels.

5. Buy in bulk. Buying larger quantities of plant-based foods can help you save money in the long run.

6. Check the expiration date. When shopping for plant-based foods, it is important to check the expiration date to ensure you are getting the freshest and safest products.

7. Read reviews. Take the time to read reviews to get an idea of what other people think of the products you are considering.

8. Ask questions. If you have any questions about the plant-based foods you are considering, don't be afraid to ask the store employees. They can provide valuable information.

9. Look for new products. Keep your eyes peeled for any new plant-based products that may be available.

10. Have fun! Plant-based shopping can be a fun and rewarding experience. Enjoy the process and don't be afraid to experiment with different items.

Finally, if you're looking to save money, try shopping at farmer's markets, ethnic grocery stores, and online sources.

These can be great places to find high-quality plant-based foods at a more affordable price.

Tips and strategies to manage food cravings

1. Eat Plenty of Whole Foods: Eating plenty of whole plant-based foods is the best way to ensure you're getting all the necessary nutrients for a healthy, balanced diet. Whole plant-based foods are packed with fiber, vitamins, minerals, and antioxidants that can help keep you feeling full and satisfied. This will aid in suppressing cravings.

2. Stock Your Kitchen with Healthy Snacks: Having plenty of healthy snacks on hand can help to prevent cravings. Pick fiber- and protein-rich snacks like nuts, seeds, and dried fruit. You can also make your own plant-based energy bars or trail mix with nuts and seeds.

3. Drink Plenty of Water: Drinking enough water throughout the day can help to keep cravings at bay. Studies have shown that even mild dehydration can lead to an increase in hunger. Keeping yourself hydrated can help to reduce cravings.

4. Get Plenty of Rest: Not getting enough sleep can lead to increased cravings. Aim for 7-9 hours of sleep each night to help keep cravings at bay.

5. Avoid Processed Foods: Processed plant-based foods, such as vegan burgers and other mock meats, often contain added salt and sugar, which can lead to cravings. It's best to avoid these foods and stick to whole plant-based foods.

6. Manage Stress: Stress can cause cravings to grow. Include stress-relieving exercises like yoga, meditation, or deep breathing in your everyday routine.

7. Move Your Body: Exercise can help to reduce stress and curb cravings. Daily physical exercise should last at least 30 minutes.

Tips and strategies for getting started

1. Start Small: When transitioning to a plant-based diet, it's best to start small and make gradual changes. Try replacing one animal-based meal with a plant-based meal each week, or start with a plant-based breakfast.

2. Focus on Whole Foods: A plant-based diet isn't just about avoiding animal products.

It's also about eating whole, unprocessed plant foods that are packed with nutrients. Focus on eating fresh fruits and vegetables, whole grains, legumes, nuts, and seeds.

3. Experiment with Plant-Based Recipes: There's no need to give up the flavors you love. Experiment with plant-based recipes that are full of flavor and nutrition. Try new dishes and ingredients to make your meals interesting.

4. Make Smart Substitutes: If you're avoiding animal products, look for plant-based alternatives. Try plant-based milks, cheeses, and yogurts in place of dairy products. There are also plant-based meat substitutes available in most grocery stores.

5. Stock Your Kitchen: Having the right ingredients on hand makes it easier to cook plant-based meals. Stock your pantry and refrigerator with plant-based staples like beans, lentils, nuts, seeds, and whole grains.

6. Don't Forget to Supplement: Plant-based diets can be low in certain vitamins and minerals, so it's important to supplement if necessary. Find out from your doctor the supplements you might require.

7. Stay Hydrated: Drinking enough water is important for overall health, and it's especially important on a plant-based diet. Aim to consume 8 glasses of water or more each day.

8. Get Support: Making changes to your diet can be difficult, so it's important to have supportive people in your life. Join a plant-based community or find a dietitian who specializes in plant-based nutrition.

Food based mistakes to avoid

When transitioning to a plant-based diet, there are certain mistakes to avoid in order to ensure optimal nutrition.

Here are some of the most common food-based mistakes to watch out for when starting with a plant-based diet:

1. Not Eating Enough Variety: Eating a variety of plant-based foods is important for optimal nutrition. Nutritional deficits may result from consuming too much of one kind of food. Be sure to include a range of fruits, vegetables, grains, legumes, nuts, and seeds in your diet.

2. Relying on Processed Foods: Many processed foods, such as veggie burgers, are not nutrient-dense. Instead, opt for whole foods that are high in nutrition such as legumes, nuts, seeds, and fresh fruits and vegetables.

3. Not Eating Enough Protein: Protein is an essential part of a healthy diet. Plant-based proteins such as beans, lentils, nuts, and seeds can provide the necessary amount of protein needed.

4. Not Eating Enough Healthy Fats: Plant-based sources of healthy fats, such as avocado, olive oil, nuts, and seeds, are important for a balanced diet.

5. Not Eating Enough Calcium: Dairy products are a major source of calcium, which is important for bone health. To get enough calcium on a plant-based diet, be sure to include foods such as leafy greens, nuts, seeds, and fortified plant-based milks.

By avoiding these common food-based mistakes, you can ensure that you are getting the nutrition you need from your plant-based diet.

CHAPTER 4

Breakfast

1. Coconut Oatmeal with Berries

Ingredients:

- Half (1/2) cup rolled oats

- Quarter (1/4) teaspoon ground cinnamon

- Quarter (1/4) teaspoon pure vanilla extract

- Quarter (1/4) cup unsweetened coconut flakes

- Quarter (1/4) cup unsweetened almond milk

- Quarter (1/4) cup mixed berries

Instructions:

-Bring a medium pot with 1 cup of water to a boil.

-Adjust heat to a low simmer and stir in the oats, cinnamon, and vanilla.

-Coconut flakes and almond milk are added; the mixture is cooked for 5 minutes while being stirred occasionally.

-Take the dish off the heat and add the berries.

-Serve hot.

Nutritional Facts:

Calories: 241, Fat: 8.4g, Carbohydrates: 35g, Protein: 5.9g, Fiber: 4.4g

Prep Time: 10 minutes

2. Avocado Toast

Ingredients:

- One (1) whole grain slice of toast

- Half (1/2) ripe avocado

-Juice of half (1/2) lemon

- Quarter (1/4) teaspoon sea salt

Instructions:

-Bread should be gently toasted.

-Avocado should be mashed before being put over toast.

-Sprinkle salt on top and squeeze some lemon juice over it.

-Enjoy.

Nutritional Facts:

Calories: 154, Fat: 8.4g, Carbohydrates: 17.4g, Protein: 3.4g, Fiber: 4.4g

Prep Time: 5 minutes

3. Chia Seed Pudding

Ingredients:

- Quarter (1/4) cup chia seeds

- One (1) cup unsweetened almond milk

- Half (1/2) teaspoon pure vanilla extract

- Half (1/2) teaspoon ground cinnamon

- One (1) tablespoon maple syrup

- Quarter (1/4) cup fresh or frozen berries

Instructions:

-In a medium bowl, whisk together the chia seeds, almond milk, vanilla, cinnamon, and maple syrup.

-Overnight in the refrigerator, cover the bowl.

-Stir the pudding and sprinkle berries over top in the morning.

Nutritional Facts:

Calories: 237, Fat: 8.6g, Carbohydrates: 28.2g, Protein: 7.2g, Fiber: 9.3g

Prep Time: 10 minutes (plus overnight soaking time)

4. Banana-Cocoa Smoothie

Ingredients:

- One (1) banana

- Half (1/2) cup almond milk

- Quarter (1/4) cup plain Greek yogurt

- One (1) tablespoon cocoa powder

- Half (1/2) teaspoon pure vanilla extract

Instructions:

-Blend all the ingredients together in a blender until they are completely smooth.

-Pour into a glass.

-Enjoy

Nutritional Facts:

Calories: 170, Fat: 4.8g, Carbohydrates: 25.3g, Protein: 8.8g, Fiber: 3.5g

Prep Time: 5 minutes

5. Tofu Scramble

Ingredients:

- One (1) tablespoon olive oil

- Half (1/2) cup diced onion

- Half (1/2) cup diced red bell pepper

- Half (1/2) cup diced mushrooms

- Half (1/2) teaspoon garlic powder

- Half (1/2) teaspoon turmeric

- Half (1/2) teaspoon cumin

- Quarter (1/4) teaspoon black pepper

- Quarter (1/4) teaspoon sea salt

- Half (1/2) block extra-firm tofu, crumbled

- Quarter (1/4) cup chopped fresh parsley

Instructions:

-In a big skillet over medium heat, heat the oil

-Add the onion, bell pepper, and mushrooms and cook for approximately 5 minutes, or until softened

-Stir in the garlic powder, turmeric, cumin, black pepper, salt and mix to combine.

-Add the tofu and simmer for 5 minutes while stirring occasionally.

-Add the parsley and continue to simmer for a few more minutes.

-Serve hot.

Nutritional Facts:

Calories: 152, Fat: 8.9g, Carbohydrates: 9.3g, Protein: 9.7g, Fiber: 3.2g

Prep Time: 15 minutes

6. Apple-Cinnamon Overnight Oats

Ingredients:

- Half (1/2) cup rolled oats

- Half (1/2) cup unsweetened almond milk

- Quarter (1/4) teaspoon ground cinnamon

- Quarter (1/4) teaspoon pure vanilla extract

- Quarter (1/4) cup diced apple

- One (1) tablespoon maple syrup

Instructions:

-In a small bowl, whisk together the oats, almond milk, cinnamon, and vanilla.

-Add the maple syrup and apple dice, then whisk to incorporate.

-The dish should be covered and refrigerate overnight

Add more apple dice to the top in the morning, if preferred.

Nutritional Facts:

Calories: 178, Fat: 3.3g, Carbohydrates: 34.3g, Protein: 3.3g, Fiber: 4.6g

Prep Time: 5 minutes (plus overnight soaking time)

7. Quinoa Power Bowl

Ingredients:

- Half (1/2) cup cooked quinoa

- Half (1/2) cup cooked black beans

- Quarter (1/4) cup diced red bell pepper

- Quarter (1/4) cup diced red onion

- Quarter (1/4) cup diced cucumber

- Two (2) tablespoons chopped fresh parsley

- Two (2) tablespoons freshly squeezed lemon juice

- Quarter (1/4) teaspoon sea salt

Instructions:

-In a medium bowl, add all the ingredients and whisk to blend.

– Serve chilled or at room temperature.

Nutritional Facts:

Calories: 177, Fat: 2.3g, Carbohydrates: 31.5g, Protein: 7.4g, Fiber: 6.5g

Prep Time: 10 minutes

8. Acai Bowl

Ingredients:

- Half (1/2) cup frozen acai berries

- Half (1/2) cup unsweetened almond milk

- Half (1/2) banana

- Quarter (1/4) cup frozen blueberries

- One (1) tablespoon chia seeds

- One (1) tablespoon hemp hearts

Instructions:

-Place the acai berries, banana, and almond milk in a blender and process until smooth.

-Place the mixture in a bowl and garnish with hemp hearts, chia seeds, and blueberries.

-Enjoy.

Nutritional Facts:

Calories: 227, Fat: 8.8g, Carbohydrates: 32.9g, Protein: 7.8g, Fiber: 8.6g

Prep Time: 5 minutes

9. Sweet Potato Toast

Ingredients:

- Half (1/2) sweet potato

- One (1) tablespoon almond butter

- Quarter (1/4) teaspoon ground cinnamon

- Quarter (1/4) teaspoon pure vanilla extract

Instructions:

-Cut the sweet potato into paper-thin pieces.

-Brown the slices on both sides in the oven.

-Sprinkle cinnamon and vanilla on top after spreading almond butter.

-Enjoy.

Nutritional Facts:

Calories: 157, Fat: 8.5g, Carbohydrates: 17.2g, Protein: 3.2g, Fiber: 3.3g

Prep Time: 10 minutes

10. Fruit and Nut Granola

Ingredients:

- Half (1/2) cup rolled oats

- Quarter (1/4) cup chopped almonds

- Quarter (1/4) cup chopped walnuts

- Quarter (1/4) cup unsweetened coconut flakes

- Quarter (1/4) teaspoon ground cinnamon

- Quarter (1/4) teaspoon sea salt

- Two (2) tablespoons maple syrup

- Quarter (1/4) cup diced dried fruit such as apricots, dates, or raisins

Instructions:

-Set oven temperature to 350°F.

-In a medium bowl, whisk together the oats, almonds, walnuts, coconut flakes, cinnamon, and salt.

-Add the maple syrup and diced fruit.

-Spread the mixture on a baking sheet, bake for 15 minutes, stirring once or twice.

-Take the food out of the oven and allow it cool fully before serving.

Nutritional Facts:

Calories: 217, Fat: 10.7g, Carbohydrates: 25.6g, Protein: 5.7g, Fiber: 4.1g

Prep Time: 20 minutes

11. Overnight Chia Pudding

Ingredients:

- Quarter (1/4) cup chia seeds

- One (1) cup unsweetened almond milk

- One (1) teaspoon pure maple syrup

- Quarter (1/4) teaspoon pure vanilla extract

- Quarter (1/4) teaspoon ground cinnamon

- Quarter (1/4) cup mixed berries

Instructions:

In a medium bowl, whisk together the chia seeds, almond milk, maple syrup, vanilla, and cinnamon.

-The dish should be covered and refrigerate overnight

-Stir the pudding in the morning, then sprinkle some berries on top.

Nutritional Facts:

Calories: 246, Fat: 8.8g, Carbohydrates: 31.6g, Protein: 7.3g, Fiber: 9.4g

Prep Time: 10 minutes (plus the overnight soaking time)

12. Vegan French Toast

Ingredients:

- Two (2) slices whole grain bread

- Half (1/2) cup unsweetened almond milk

- Quarter (1/4) teaspoon ground cinnamon

- Quarter (1/4) teaspoon pure vanilla extract

- Quarter (1/4) teaspoon ground nutmeg

- One (1) tablespoon maple syrup

Instructions:

-In a small dish, mix the almond milk, cinnamon, vanilla, and nutmeg.

-Every piece of bread should be dipped in the sauce and let to soak for a few minutes.

-Spray cooking spray into a big skillet and heat over medium heat.

-In the skillet, add the moistened bread, and cook for a few minutes on each side, or until golden brown.

-Add maple syrup on top, Enjoy.

Nutritional Facts:

Calories: 181, Fat: 3.4g, Carbohydrates: 29.4g, Protein: 5.7g, Fiber: 2.9g

Prep Time: 10 minutes

13. Savory Oatmeal

Ingredients:

- Half (1/2) cup rolled oats

- Quarter (1/4) teaspoon sea salt

- Quarter (1/4) teaspoon ground black pepper

- Quarter (1/4) teaspoon garlic powder

- Quarter (1/4) teaspoon onion powder

- Quarter (1/4) cup unsweetened almond milk

- One (1) tablespoon nutritional yeast

Instructions:

-Boil one cup of water in a medium saucepan.

-Raise the temperature to a low simmer and add the oats, salt, pepper, garlic powder, and onion powder.

-After include the almond milk, cook for five minutes while stirring occasionally.

-Turn of the heat and add the nutritional yeast.

-Serve hot.

Nutritional Facts:

Calories: 171, Fat: 4.3g, Carbohydrates: 27.8g, Protein: 6.5g, Fiber: 4.1g

Prep Time: 10 minutes

14. Banana Oat Pancakes

Ingredients:

- Half (1/2) cup rolled oats

- Quarter (1/4) teaspoon baking powder

- Quarter (1/4) teaspoon ground cinnamon

- Quarter (1/4) cup mashed banana

- Quarter (1/4) cup unsweetened almond milk

Instructions:

-In a larger bowl, whisk together the oats, cinnamon, and baking powder.

-Continue stirring after adding the mashed banana and almond milk.

-Use cooking spray to pre-heat a sizable skillet over medium heat.

-Using a measuring cup with a 1/4 cup capacity, pour the batter onto the skillet.

-Cook until golden brown, a few minutes per side.

-If desired, put more banana puree over top.

Nutritional Facts:

Calories: 146, Fat: 2.6g, Carbohydrates: 27.9g, Protein: 4.2g, Fiber: 4.1g

Prep Time: 10 minutes

15. PB&J Smoothie

Ingredients:

- One (1) banana

- Half (1/2) cup unsweetened almond milk

- Two (2) tablespoons peanut butter

- One (1) tablespoon chia seeds

- One (1) tablespoon pure maple syrup

- Quarter (1/4) cup frozen mixed berries

Instructions:

-Banana, almond milk, peanut butter, chia seeds, and maple syrup should all be combined in a blender and processed until smooth.

-Blend in the frozen berries.

-Pour into a glass, then sip.

Nutritional Facts

:Calories: 297, Fat: 14.4g, Carbohydrates: 33.1g, Protein: 9.2g, Fiber: 7.4g

Prep Time: 5 minutes

Lunch

16. Mediterranean Chickpea Salad:

Ingredients:

- One 1 (15 ounce) can chickpeas, drained and rinsed

- One (1) cup diced cucumber

- One (1) cup diced tomatoes

- Half (1/2) cup diced red onion

- Half (1/2) cup diced bell pepper

- Quarter (1/4) cup chopped fresh parsley

- Quarter (1/4) cup sliced black olives

- Two (2) tablespoons fresh lemon juice

- Two (2) tablespoons olive oil

- One (1) teaspoon dried oregano

- Salt and pepper to taste

Instructions:

-Chickpeas, cucumber, tomatoes, red onion, bell pepper, parsley, black olives, lemon juice, olive oil, and oregano should all be combined in a big bowl.

-Gently stir by tossing.

-To taste, add salt and pepper to the food.

– Serve cold or room temperature.

Nutritional facts:

Calories: 274, Fat: 13.3 g, Carbohydrates: 32.9 g, Fiber:8.6g, Protein: 8.7 g

Prep time: 10 minutes

17. Tempeh & Veggie Bowl:

Ingredients:

- One (1) teaspoon olive oil

- One 1 (8 ounce) package tempeh, diced

- Half (1/2) teaspoon dried oregano

- Quarter (1/4) teaspoon garlic powder

- Quarter (1/4) teaspoon onion powder

- Quarter (1/4) teaspoon smoked paprika

- Quarter (1/4) teaspoon ground cumin

- Quarter (1/4) teaspoon ground coriander

- Quarter (1/4) teaspoon turmeric

- Quarter (1/4) teaspoon ground black pepper

- One (1) cup diced bell pepper

- One (1) cup diced zucchini

- One (1) cup cooked brown rice

- Quarter (1/4) cup sliced black olives

-Salt to taste

Instructions:

-In a big skillet, heat the olive oil over medium-high heat.

-Add tempeh and season with oregano, cumin, coriander, black pepper, smoked paprika, garlic powder, onion powder, and turmeric. Cook for approximately 5 minutes, stirring periodically, until gently browned.

-Add the bell pepper and zucchini, and simmer for approximately 5 minutes, turning periodically, until the veggies are soft.

-Brown rice should be cooked before being added.

-Add salt to taste and toss to mix.

-Serve warm.

Nutritional facts:

Calories: 358, Fat: 13.6 g, Carbohydrates: 40.7 g,

Fiber: 7.7 g, Protein: 17.1 g

Prep time: 15 minutes

18. Lentil & Spinach Curry:

Ingredients:

- One (1) tablespoon olive oil

- One (1) small onion, diced

- Two (2) cloves garlic, minced

- One (1) tablespoon grated fresh ginger

- One (1) teaspoon ground cumin

- One (1) teaspoon ground coriander

- Quarter (1/4) teaspoon turmeric

- Quarter (1/4) teaspoon ground cinnamon

- Quarter (1/4) teaspoon cayenne pepper

- One 1 (14.5 ounce) can diced tomatoes

- One 1 (14 ounce) can coconut milk

- One 1 (15 ounce) can lentils, drained and rinsed

- Two (2) cups baby spinach

-Salt and pepper to taste

Instructions:

-In a big skillet, heat the olive oil over medium heat.

-Add the onion and garlic and simmer for about 5 minutes, stirring regularly, until tender.

-Stirring constantly for one minute, add the ginger, cumin, coriander, turmeric, cinnamon, and cayenne pepper.

-Add coconut milk and tomatoes, and then boil.

-Add lentils and spinach, and simmer, stirring periodically, for about 3 minutes, or until spinach has wilted.

-To taste, add salt and pepper to the food.

-Serve warm.

Nutritional facts:

Calories: 462, Fat: 24.3 g, Carbohydrates: 45.9 g,

Fiber: 14.7 g, Protein: 15.8 g

Prep time: 15 minutes

19. Veggie Burrito Bowl:

Ingredients:

- One (1) tablespoon olive oil

- One (1) small onion, diced

- One (1) bell pepper, diced

- Two (2) cloves garlic, minced

- One 1 (15 ounce) can black beans, drained and rinsed

- One (1) teaspoon chili powder

- One (1) teaspoon ground cumin

- Quarter (1/4) teaspoon smoked paprika

- Quarter (1/4) teaspoon ground coriander

- Quarter (1/4) teaspoon turmeric

-Salt and pepper to taste

- One (1) cup cooked brown rice

- Quarter (1/4) cup diced tomatoes

- Quarter (1/4) cup diced avocado

- Quarter (1/4) cup diced red onion

- Two (2) tablespoons chopped fresh cilantro

- Two (2) tablespoons sliced black olives

Instructions:

-In a big skillet, heat the olive oil over medium-high heat.

-Add the onion, bell pepper and garlic and simmer for 5 minutes, stirring occasionally, until softened

-Add black beans, chili powder, cumin, smoked paprika, coriander and turmeric and simmer for additional 1 minute, stirring.

-To taste, add salt and pepper to the food.

-Shared the cooked rice into four bowls.

-Top all the bowls with bean mixture, tomatoes, avocado, red onion, cilantro and olives.

-Serve warm.

Nutritional facts:

Calories: 471, Fat: 15.3 g , Carbohydrates: 66.2 g,

Fiber: 17.7 g, Protein: 18.6 g

Prep time: 15 minutes

20. Zucchini Noodle Bowl:

Ingredients:

- One (1) tablespoon olive oil

- One (1) small onion, diced

- Two (2) cloves garlic, minced

- One (1) teaspoon dried oregano

- Half (1/2) teaspoon ground cumin

- Quarter (1/4) teaspoon smoked paprika

- Quarter (1/4) teaspoon ground turmeric

- Quarter (1/4) teaspoon ground coriander

- Quarter (1/4) teaspoon ground black pepper

- Two (2) cups vegetable broth

- One 1 (14.5 ounce) can diced tomatoes

- Two (2) medium zucchini, spiralized

-Salt and pepper to taste

Instructions:

-In a big skillet, heat the olive oil over medium-high heat.

-Add the onion and garlic and simmer for 5 minutes, stirring occasionally, until softened.

-Add oregano, cumin, paprika, turmeric, coriander and black pepper and simmer for additional 1 minute, stirring.

-Add vegetable broth and tomatoes and bring to a simmer.

-Add the zucchini noodles and simmer for 5 minutes, stirring occasionally, until tender.

-To taste, add salt and pepper to the food.

-Serve warm.

Nutritional facts:

Calories: 211, Fat: 8.8 g, Carbohydrates: 27.4 g,

Fiber: 5.4 g, Protein: 7.7 g

Prep time: 10 minutes

21. Quinoa & Veggie Stir Fry:

Ingredients:

- One (1) tablespoon olive oil

- One (1) small onion, diced

- Two (2) cloves garlic, minced

- One (1) teaspoon grated fresh ginger

- Half (1/2) teaspoon ground cumin

- Quarter (1/4) teaspoon ground coriander

- Quarter (1/4) teaspoon turmeric

- Quarter (1/4) teaspoon smoked paprika

- Quarter (1/4) teaspoon ground black pepper

- One (1) cup diced bell pepper

- One (1) cup diced zucchini

- One (1) cup cooked quinoa

- Quarter (1/4) cup chopped fresh parsley

-Salt and pepper to taste

Instructions:

-In a big skillet, heat the olive oil over medium-high heat.

-Add the onion and garlic and simmer for 5 minutes, stirring occasionally, until softened.

-Add the ginger, cumin, coriander, turmeric, smoked paprika and black pepper and simmer for additional 1 minute, stirring.

-Add the bell pepper and zucchini and simmer for another 5 minutes, stirring occasionally, until vegetables are tender.

-Add the cooked quinoa, parsley

-To taste, add salt and pepper to the food.

-Serve warm.

Nutritional facts:

Calories: 304, Fat: 11.2 g, Carbohydrates: 36.6 g,

Fiber: 5.8 g, Protein: 10.2 g

Prep time: 15 minutes

22. Cauliflower & Potato Curry:

Ingredients:

- One (1) tablespoon olive oil

- One (1) small onion, diced

- Two (2) cloves garlic, minced

- One (1) tablespoon grated fresh ginger

- One (1) teaspoon ground cumin

- Half (1/2) teaspoon ground coriander

- Quarter (1/4) teaspoon turmeric

- Quarter (1/4) teaspoon ground black pepper

- Quarter (1/4) teaspoon cayenne pepper

- One 1 (14.5 ounce) can coconut milk

- One (1) head cauliflower, cut into florets

- Two (2) medium potatoes, cubed

- Quarter (1/4) cup chopped fresh cilantro

-Salt and pepper to taste

Instructions:

-In a big skillet, heat the olive oil over medium-high heat.

-Add the onion and garlic and simmer for 5 minutes, stirring occasionally, until softened.

-Add ginger, cumin, coriander, turmeric, black pepper and cayenne pepper and simmer for additional 1 minute, stirring.

-Add coconut milk and then boil.

-Add cauliflower and potatoes and simmer for another 10 minutes, stirring occasionally, until vegetables are tender.

-Add cilantro and season with salt and pepper to taste.

-Serve warm.

Nutritional facts:

Calories: 398, Fat: 22.3 g, Carbohydrates: 38.6 g,

Fiber: 9.8 g, Protein: 10.7 g

Prep time: 15 minutes

23. Roasted Sweet Potato & Kale Bowl:

Ingredients:

- Two (2) sweet potatoes, cubed

- One (1) tablespoon olive oil

- One (1) teaspoon smoked paprika

- Half (1/2) teaspoon ground cumin

- Quarter (1/4) teaspoon garlic powder

- Quarter (1/4) teaspoon ground coriander

- Quarter (1/4) teaspoon ground black pepper

- Two (2) cups chopped kale

- Half (1/2) cup cooked quinoa

- Quarter (1/4) cup diced tomatoes

- Quarter (1/4) cup diced red onion

- Two (2) tablespoons sliced black olives

-Salt and pepper to taste

Instructions:

-Set the oven temperature to 400°F.

-In a medium bowl, put together sweet potatoes, olive oil, smoked paprika, cumin, garlic powder, coriander and black pepper. Toss to coat.

-Spread the mixture on a baking sheet and roast in preheated oven for 20 minutes, or until tender.

-In a medium bowl, combine kale, quinoa, tomatoes, red onion and olives.

-Add the roasted sweet potatoes and mix together.

-To taste, add salt and pepper

-Serve warm.

Nutritional facts:

Calories: 313, Fat: 10.2 g, Carbohydrates: 47.3 g,

Fiber: 7.7 g, Protein: 7.9 g

Prep time: 15 minutes

24. Broccoli & Tofu Stir Fry:

Ingredients:

- One (1) tablespoon olive oil

- One (1) small onion, diced

- Two (2) cloves garlic, minced

- One (1) teaspoon grated fresh ginger

- Half (1/2) teaspoon ground cumin

- Quarter (1/4) teaspoon ground coriander

- Quarter (1/4) teaspoon turmeric

- Quarter (1/4) teaspoon smoked paprika

- Quarter (1/4) teaspoon ground black pepper

- One 1 (14 ounce) package extra-firm tofu, cubed

- Two (2) cups broccoli florets

- Quarter (1/4) cup vegetable broth

- Two (2) tablespoons soy sauce

- Two (2) tablespoons chopped fresh cilantro

-Salt and pepper to taste

Instructions:

-In a big skillet, heat the olive oil over medium-high heat.

-Add the onion and garlic and simmer for 5 minutes, stirring occasionally, until softened.

-Add ginger, cumin, coriander, turmeric, smoked paprika and black pepper and simmer for additional 1 minute, stirring.

-Add the tofu and broccoli and simmer for another 5 minutes, stirring occasionally, until broccoli is tender.

-Add the vegetable broth, soy sauce and cilantro and simmer for additional 2 minutes, stirring, until heated through.

-To taste, add salt and pepper

-Serve warm.

Nutritional facts:

Calories: 295, Fat: 14.2 g, Carbohydrates: 19.7 g,

Fiber: 5.4 g, Protein: 20.7 g

Prep time: 10 minutes

25. Eggplant & Chickpea Curry:

Ingredients:

- One (1) tablespoon olive oil

- One (1) small onion, diced

- Two (2) cloves garlic, minced

- One (1) teaspoon grated fresh ginger

- One (1) teaspoon ground cumin

- Half (1/2) teaspoon ground coriander

- Quarter (1/4) teaspoon turmeric

- Quarter (1/4) teaspoon ground black pepper

- Quarter (1/4) teaspoon cayenne pepper

- One 1 (14.5 ounce) can diced tomatoes

- One 1 (14 ounce) can coconut milk

- One (1) medium eggplant, cubed

- One 1 (15 ounce) can chickpeas, drained and rinsed

- Two (2) tablespoons chopped fresh cilantro

-Salt and pepper to taste

Instructions:

-In a big skillet, heat the olive oil over medium-high heat.

-Add the onion and garlic and simmer for 5 minutes, stirring occasionally, until softened.

-Add ginger, cumin, coriander, turmeric, black pepper and cayenne pepper and simmer for additional 1 minute, stirring.

-Stir in the tomatoes and coconut milk and bring to a simmer.

-Add eggplant and chickpeas and simmer for another 10 minutes, stirring occasionally, until eggplant is tender.

-Add cilantro and season with salt and pepper to taste.

-Serve warm.

Nutritional facts:

Calories: 463, Fat: 25.7 g, Carbohydrates: 47.1 g

Fiber: 14.2 g, Protein: 13.2 g

Prep time: 15 minutes

26. Hummus Wrap:

Ingredients:

- Two (2) whole wheat tortillas

- Quarter (1/4) cup hummus

- Quarter (1/4) cup diced bell pepper

- Quarter (1/4) cup diced cucumber

- Quarter (1/4) cup diced tomatoes

- Quarter (1/4) cup shredded lettuce

- Two (2) tablespoons sliced black olives

Instructions:

-Gradually spread hummus on each tortilla.

-Bell pepper, cucumber, tomatoes, lettuce and olives should be added to the top of each tortilla.

-Gently roll each tortilla into a wrap.

-Cut each wraps in half and serve.

Nutritional facts:

Calories: 263, Fat: 10 g, Carbohydrates: 35.5 g

Fiber: 8.1 g, Protein: 10.3 g

Prep time: 10 minutes

27. Lentil Soup:

Ingredients:

- One (1) tablespoon olive oil

- One (1) small onion, diced

- Two (2) cloves garlic, minced

- One (1) teaspoon grated fresh ginger

- One (1) teaspoon ground cumin

- Half (1/2) teaspoon ground coriander

- Quarter (1/4) teaspoon turmeric

- Quarter (1/4) teaspoon smoked paprika

- Quarter (1/4) teaspoon ground black pepper

- Quarter (1/4) teaspoon cayenne pepper

- Six (6) cups vegetable broth

- One 1 (15 ounce) can lentils, drained and rinsed

- One 1 (14.5 ounce) can diced tomatoes

- Two (2) cups baby spinach

-Salt and pepper to taste

Instructions:

-In a big skillet, heat the olive oil over medium-high heat.

-Add the onion and garlic and simmer for 5 minutes, stirring occasionally, until softened.

-Add ginger, cumin, coriander, turmeric, smoked paprika, black pepper and cayenne pepper and simmer for additional 1 minute, stirring.

-Add vegetable broth and bring to a boil.

-Add the lentils and tomatoes and simmer for another 5 minutes, stirring occasionally, until heated through.

-Stir in spinach and season with salt and pepper to taste.

-Serve warm.

Nutritional facts:

Calories: 376, Fat: 8.3 g, Carbohydrates: 54 g,

Fiber: 21.3 g, Protein: 19.4 g

Prep time: 15 minutes

28. Avocado & Pinto Bean Burrito:

Ingredients:

- Two (2) whole wheat tortillas

- Half (1/2) cup cooked pinto beans

- Quarter (1/4) cup diced tomatoes

- Quarter (1/4) cup diced red onion

- Quarter (1/4) cup diced avocado

- Quarter (1/4) cup shredded lettuce

- Two (2) tablespoons chopped fresh cilantro

Instructions:

-Gently spread pinto beans on each tortilla.

-Tomatoes, red onion, avocado, lettuce and cilantro should be added to top each tortilla.

3. Roll each tortilla into a burrito.

4. Cut burritos in half and serve.

Nutritional facts:

Calories: 314, Fat: 10.5 g, Carbohydrates: 40.6 g,

Fiber: 9.5 g, Protein: 12 g

Prep time: 10 minutes

29. Baked Sweet Potato & Black Bean Burrito:

Ingredients:

- Two (2) large sweet potatoes, baked

- One (1) tablespoon olive oil

- One (1) small onion, diced

- Two (2) cloves garlic, minced

- One (1) teaspoon ground cumin

- Half (1/2) teaspoon ground coriander

- Quarter (1/4) teaspoon smoked paprika

- Quarter (1/4) teaspoon turmeric

- Quarter (1/4) teaspoon chili powder

- Quarter (1/4) teaspoon sea salt

- One 1 (15-ounce) can black beans, drained and rinsed

- Two (2) cups fresh spinach, chopped

- Two (2) tablespoons fresh lime juice

- Four (4) large whole wheat tortillas

Instructions:

-Set the oven temperature to 375°F.

-Line the baking sheet with a parchment paper.

-Spread the sweet potatoes out on a baking sheet, and bake for 45 to 50 minutes, or until fork-tender. Remove from oven once finished and allow to cool.

-In a big skillet, heat the olive oil over medium-high heat, add the onion and simmer for 5 minutes.

-Include salt, turmeric, chili powder, cumin, coriander, smoked paprika, and cumin. Simmer for additional 1 minute.

-Stir in black beans and then simmer for another 5 minutes.

-After the spinach has wilted, add lime juice and simmer for a further 3 minutes.

-Halve sweet potatoes lengthwise. Scoop out the flesh, then add it to the skillet. With a fork, mash the avocado and combine with the remaining ingredients.

-Microwave tortillas for 30 seconds to reheat.

-Place a portion of the sweet potato mixture on each tortilla, and then roll.

-You can either serve it right away or wrap it in foil and keep it in the fridge for up to three days.

Nutritional Facts:

Calories: 300 , Carbohydrates: 40 g , Protein: 10 g ,

Fat: 10 g , Fiber: 8 g , Sugar: 6 g

Prep Time: 1hr 15 minutes

30. Zucchini Noodle Bowl:

Ingredients:

- One (1) tablespoon olive oil

- One (1) small onion, diced

- Three (3) cloves garlic, minced

- Two (2) zucchinis, spiralized

- One (1) red bell pepper, diced

- Quarter (1/4) teaspoon sea salt

- Quarter (1/4) teaspoon black pepper

- Quarter (1/4) teaspoon paprika

- Quarter (1/4) teaspoon garlic powder

- One 1 (15-ounce) can black beans, drained and rinsed

- One 1 (14.5-ounce) can diced tomatoes

- Quarter (1/4) cup fresh cilantro, chopped

- Quarter (1/4) cup fresh parsley, chopped

- Quarter (1/4) cup toasted pumpkin seeds

Instructions:

-In a big skillet, heat the olive oil over medium-high heat.

-Add the onion and garlic and simmer for 5 minutes.

-Add zucchini noodles, bell pepper, salt, pepper, paprika, and garlic powder. And simmer for additional 5 minutes or until zucchini is tender.

-Add the black beans, tomatoes, cilantro, and parsley, and simmer for another 5 minutes.

-Add pumpkin seeds on top and divide the zucchini noodle mixture into two dishes.

-Immediately serve, or keep chilled for up to three days.

Nutritional Facts:

Calories: 310 , Carbohydrates: 33 g , Protein: 12 g,

Fat: 15 g , Fiber: 9 g , Sugar: 8 g

Prep Time: 20 minutes

Dinner

31. Baked Portobello Mushrooms with Polenta

Ingredients:

- Four (4) large portobello mushrooms

- One (1) cup cooked polenta

- Two (2) tablespoons olive oil

- One (1) teaspoon garlic powder

- Salt and pepper, to taste

- Quarter (1/4) cup nutritional yeast

Instructions:

-Set the oven temperature to 375F.

-Clean the mushrooms and cut off the stems.

-Place the polenta that has been prepared on top of the mushrooms in the baking dish.

-Drizzle olive oil over the mushrooms and then season with salt, pepper, and garlic powder.

-Cook for 25 minutes in a preheated oven.

-Add nutritional yeast and serve.

Nutrition Facts:

Calories: 294, Fat: 15g, Carbohydrates: 30g, Protein: 11g,

Fiber: 6g, Sugar: 1g

Prep Time: 35 minutes

32. Roasted Vegetable Quinoa Bowl

Ingredients:

- One (1) cup cooked quinoa,

- One (1) cup diced carrots

- One (1) cup diced red bell peppers

- One (1) cup diced zucchini

- Half (1/2) cup diced onion

- Two (2) tablespoons olive oil

- One (1) teaspoon garlic powder

- Salt and pepper, to taste

Instructions:

-Set the oven temperature to 375F.

-Add olive oil to a big bowl and add all the veggies.

-Add salt, pepper, and garlic powder, and stir to blend.

-Arrange the veggies on a baking sheet in an equal layer.

-Bake for 25 minutes in a preheated oven, stirring halfway through.

-Serve the veggies over cooked quinoa.

Nutrition Facts:

Calories: 238, Fat: 8g, Carbohydrates: 34g, Protein: 7g

Fiber: 6g, Sugar: 5g

Prep Time: 35 minutes

33. Lentil Fajita Bowls

Ingredients:

- Two (2) cups cooked lentils

- One (1) red bell pepper, sliced

- One (1) yellow bell pepper, sliced

- One (1) green bell pepper, sliced

- One (1) onion, sliced

- Two (2) tablespoons olive oil

- One (1) teaspoon chili powder

- One (1) teaspoon garlic powder

- Salt and pepper, to taste

Instructions:

-Set the oven temperature to 375F.

-Add olive oil to a big bowl and add all the veggies.

-Add chili powder, garlic powder, salt, and pepper and stir to blend.

-Arrange the vegetables on a baking sheet equal layer.

-Bake for 25 minutes in a preheated oven, stirring halfway through.

-Serve the cooked lentils topped with roasted vegetables.

Nutrition Facts:

Calories: 248, Fat: 8g, Carbohydrates: 33g, Protein: 11g

Fiber: 10g, Sugar: 7g

Prep Time: 35 minutes

34. Chickpea Veggie Burgers

Ingredients:

- One (1) can chickpeas, drained and rinsed

- Half (1/2) cup rolled oats

- Half (1/4) cup diced onion

- Half (1/4) cup diced red bell pepper

- Half (1/4) cup diced carrot

- Two (2) tablespoons olive oil

- One (1) teaspoon garlic powder

- Salt and pepper, to taste

Instructions:

-Set the oven temperature to 375F.

-Place chickpeas in a large bowl and mashed with a fork.

-Add the carrot, onion, bell pepper, and oats; stir to incorporate.

-Create 4 patties out of the mixture, and set them on a baking pan.

-Sprinkle salt, pepper, and garlic powder over the burgers after drizzling them with olive oil.

-Bake for 20 minutes in a preheated oven, flipping halfway through.

Nutrition Facts:

Calories: 265, Fat: 8g, Carbohydrates: 36g, Protein: 9g

Fiber: 8g, Sugar: 4g

Prep Time: 30 minutes

35. Coconut Curry Noodle Bowl

Ingredients:

- Two (2) cups cooked noodles

- One (1) cup diced carrots

- One (1) cup diced red bell peppers

- One (1) cup diced zucchini

- Half (1/2) cup diced onion

- One (1) can coconut milk

- One (1) tablespoon curry powder

- One (1) teaspoon garlic powder

- Salt and pepper, to taste

Instructions:

-In a big skillet, heat the olive oil over medium-high heat.

-Add the carrots, bell peppers, zucchini, onion, and simmer for 5 minutes, stirring occasionally.

-Add the coconut milk and whisk in the curry powder, garlic powder, salt, and pepper.

-Simmer for 10 minutes while stirring periodically.

-Add the prepared noodles and simmer for 5 minutes.

-Serve warm.

Nutrition Facts:

Calories: 306, Fat: 17g, Carbohydrates: 32g, Protein: 7g

Fiber: 6g, Sugar: 6g

Prep Time: 30 minutes

36. Stuffed Sweet Potatoes

Ingredients:

- Four (4) small sweet potatoes

- One (1) can black beans, drained and rinsed

- Half (1/2) cup corn

- Quarter (1/4) cup diced red bell pepper

- Two (2) tablespoons olive oil

- One (1) teaspoon chili powder

- One (1) teaspoon garlic powder

- Salt and pepper, to taste

Instructions:

-Set the oven temperature to 375F.

-Arrange sweet potatoes on a baking sheet and bake for 45 minutes in a preheated oven.

-Combine the beans, corn, bell pepper, olive oil, garlic powder, chili powder, salt, and pepper in a medium bowl.

-Cut sweet potatoes in half and fill with bean mixture when they are finished cooking.

-Put the oven back on and bake for another 10 minutes.

-Serve warm.

Nutrition Facts:

Calories: 275, Fat: 8g, Carbohydrates: 42g, Protein: 9g

Fiber: 9g, Sugar: 5g

Prep Time: 1 hour 5 minutes

37. Lentil Stuffed Peppers

Ingredients:

- Four (4) bell peppers

- One (1) cup cooked lentils

- Half (1/2) cup diced onion

- Quarter (1/4) cup diced celery

- Two (2) tablespoons olive oil

- One (1) teaspoon garlic powder

- Salt and pepper, to taste

Instructions:

-Set the oven temperature to 375F.

-Cut the bell peppers' tops off and scoop out the seeds.

-Combine the lentils, onion, celery, olive oil, garlic powder, salt, and pepper in a medium bowl.

-Insert the lentil mixture into each bell pepper.

-Put the filled peppers on a baking tray and bake for 25 minutes in a preheated oven.

-Serve warm.

Nutrition Facts:

Calories: 217, Fat: 7g, Carbohydrates: 29g, Protein: 10g

Fiber: 11g, Sugar: 8g

Prep Time: 35 minutes

38. Roasted Cauliflower Tacos

Ingredients:

- One (1) head cauliflower

- Two (2) tablespoons olive oil

- One (1) teaspoon chili powder

- One (1) teaspoon garlic powder

- Salt and pepper, to taste

- Eight (8) small flour tortillas

- Quarter (1/4) cup diced onion

- Quarter (1/4) cup diced tomatoes

- Quarter (1/4) cup diced cucumber

Instructions:

-Set the oven temperature to 375F.

-Separate the florets of cauliflower and spread them out on
a baking pan.

-Sprinkle with salt, pepper, garlic powder, chili powder, and olive oil.

-Bake for 25 minutes while stirring halfway through in a preheated oven.

-Use a medium-hot pan to warm up the tortillas.

-Each tortilla should be stuffed with roasted cauliflower, onion, tomatoes, and cucumber before tacos are ready to be assembled.

-Serve warm.

Nutrition Facts:

Calories: 189, Fat: 7g, Carbohydrates: 27g, Protein: 5g

Fiber: 5g, Sugar: 4g

Prep Time: 35 minutes

39. Eggplant Parmesan

Ingredients:

- Two (2) eggplants, sliced

- Two (2) tablespoons olive oil

- One (1) teaspoon garlic powder

- Salt and pepper, to taste

- Half (1/2) cup marinara sauce

- Quarter (1/4) cup nutritional yeast

Instructions:

-Set the oven temperature to 375F.

-Arrange the slices of eggplant on a baking sheet and sprinkle with olive oil.

-Add salt, pepper, and garlic powder to taste.

-Bake for 25 minutes in a preheated oven, turning the pan halfway through.

-Drizzle nutritional yeast over eggplant slices after spreading marinara sauce over them.

-Bake for additional 10 minutes.

-Serve warm.

Nutrition Facts:

Calories: 227, Fat: 10g, Carbohydrates: 30g, Protein: 9g

Fiber: 9g, Sugar: 13g

Prep Time: 45 minutes

40. Stuffed Acorn Squash

Ingredients:

- Two (2) acorn squash, halved and seeds removed

- One (1) cup cooked quinoa

- Quarter (1/4) cup diced red onion

- Quarter (1/4) cup diced red bell pepper

- Two (2) tablespoons olive oil

- One (1) teaspoon garlic powder

- Salt and pepper, to taste

Instructions:

-Set the oven temperature to 375F.

-Arrange the squash halves on a baking sheet and bake for 25 minutes in a preheated oven.

-Combine the quinoa, onion, bell pepper, olive oil, garlic powder, salt, and pepper in a medium bowl.

-Remove the baked squash from the oven and stuff it with the quinoa mixture.

-Put the dish back in the oven and bake it for 10 more minutes.

-Serve warm.

Nutrition Facts:

Calories: 270, Fat: 8g, Carbohydrates: 42g, Protein: 8g

Fiber: 8g, Sugar: 8g

Prep Time: 45 minutes

41. Baked Tofu with Rice

Ingredients:

- One (1) block extra-firm tofu, cubed

- One (1) cup cooked white rice

- Two (2) tablespoons olive oil

- One (1) teaspoon garlic powder

- Salt and pepper, to taste

- Quarter (1/4) cup nutritional yeast

Instructions:

-Set the oven temperature to 375F.

-Spread some olive oil over the tofu cubes and place them on a baking sheet.

-Add salt, pepper, and garlic powder to taste.

-Bake for 25 minutes in a preheated oven while stirring once.

-Spoon nutritional yeast on top of the tofu before serving it with cooked white rice

Nutrition Facts:

Calories: 294, Fat: 15g, Carbohydrates: 30g, Protein: 11g

Fiber: 6g, Sugar: 1g

Prep Time: 35 minutes

42. Veggie Noodle Stir Fry

Ingredients:

- Two (2) cups cooked noodles

- One (1) cup diced carrots

- One (1) cup diced red bell peppers

- One (1) cup diced zucchini

- Two (2) tablespoons olive oil

- One (1) teaspoon garlic powder

- Salt and pepper, to taste

Instructions:

-In a big skillet, heat the olive oil over medium-high heat.

-Add carrots, bell peppers, zucchini, olive oil, garlic powder, salt, and pepper and simmer for 5 minutes, stirring occasionally.

-Add the cooked noodles and continue cooking for an additional five minutes.

-Serve warm.

Nutrition Facts:

Calories: 248, Fat: 8g, Carbohydrates: 34g, Protein: 7g

Fiber: 6g, Sugar: 5g

Prep Time: 20 minutes

43. Ratatouille

Ingredients:

- One (1) eggplant, diced

- One (1) zucchini, diced

- One (1) yellow squash, diced

- One (1) red bell pepper, diced

- One (1) onion, diced

- Two (2) tablespoons olive oil

- One (1) teaspoon garlic powder

- Salt and pepper, to taste

Instructions:

-In a big skillet, heat the olive oil over medium-high heat.

-Add eggplant, zucchini, squash, bell pepper, onion, olive oil, garlic powder, salt, and pepper and simmer for 10 minutes, stirring occasionally.

-Serve warm.

Nutrition Facts:

Calories: 164, Fat: 8g, Carbohydrates: 20g, Protein: 4g,

Fiber: 7g, Sugar: 9g

Prep Time: 20 minutes

44. Baked Zucchini Fries

Ingredients:

- Three (3) zucchinis, cut into fry-shaped pieces

- Two (2) tablespoons olive oil

- One (1) teaspoon garlic powder

- Salt and pepper, to taste

- Quarter (1/4) cup nutritional yeast

Instructions:

-Set the oven temperature to 375F.

-Arrange the chunks of zucchini on a baking sheet and sprinkle with olive oil.

-Add salt, pepper, and garlic powder to taste.

-Bake for 25 minutes in a preheated oven, turning the pan halfway through.

-Top with nutritional yeast before serving.

Nutrition Facts:

Calories: 186, Fat: 10g, Carbohydrates: 18g, Protein: 9g

Fiber: 5g, Sugar: 4g

Prep Time: 35 minutes

45. Quinoa Chili

Ingredients:

- Two (2) cups cooked quinoa

- One (1) can black beans, drained and rinsed

- One (1) can diced tomatoes

- One (1) onion, diced

- One (1) red bell pepper, diced

- One (2) tablespoons olive oil

- One (1) teaspoon chili powder

- One (1) teaspoon garlic powder

- Salt and pepper, to taste

Instructions:

-In a big skillet, heat the olive oil over medium-high heat.

-Add onion, bell pepper, olive oil, chili powder, garlic powder, salt, and pepper and simmer for 5 minutes, stirring occasionally.

-Add black beans, tomatoes, and quinoa and simmer for another 10 minutes, stirring occasionally.

-Serve warm.

Nutrition Facts:

Calories: 286, Fat: 8g, Carbohydrates: 41g, Protein: 11g

Fiber: 10g, Sugar: 7g

Prep Time: 25 minutes

Snacks and Appetizer

46. Hummus and Veggie Sticks

Ingredients:

- One (1) can chickpeas, drained

- Two (2) cloves garlic, minced

- Two (2) tablespoons tahini

- One (1) tablespoon lemon juice

- Three (3) tablespoons olive oil

- Quarter (1/4) teaspoon cumin

- Quarter (1/4) teaspoon paprika

-Salt and pepper to taste

-Vegetables of your choice (e.g. celery, carrots, bell peppers, cucumber, broccoli, etc.)

Instructions:

-In a food processor, combine all ingredients (apart from the veggies) and process until smooth.

-Taste for seasoning and make any adjustments.

-Serve with your preferred chopped veggies.

Nutritional Facts:

Calories: 75 , Fat: 6 g, Carbohydrates: 5 g, Fiber: 2 g

Protein: 2 g

Prep Time: 10 minutes

47. Baked Sweet Potato Fries

Ingredients:

- Two (2) large sweet potatoes, cut into fries

- Two (2) tablespoons olive oil

- One (1) teaspoon garlic powder

- Half (1/2) teaspoon paprika

-Salt and pepper to taste

Instructions:

-Set the oven temperature to 400°F and cover baking sheet with parchment paper.

-Rub olive oil and seasonings on the sweet potatoes.

-Fries should be layered evenly on the baking pan.

-Bake for 25–30 minutes, turning once.

Nutritional Facts:

Calories: 86 , Fat: 5 g, Carbohydrates: 10 g, Fiber: 2 g

Protein: 1 g

Prep Time: 15 minutes

48. Roasted Eggplant Dip

Ingredients:

- One (1) large eggplant

- One (1) tablespoon olive oil

- One (1) garlic clove, minced

- Two (2) tablespoons tahini

- Two (2) tablespoons lemon juice

- One (1) tablespoon fresh parsley, chopped

-Salt and pepper to taste

Instructions:

-Set the oven temperature to 375°F and cover baking sheet with parchment paper.

-Halve the eggplant lengthwise, then lightly oil both sides.

-Place eggplant halves cut side down on baking sheet.

-Roast eggplant for 20 to 25 minutes, or until fork-tender and slightly browned.

-After allowing the eggplant to cool slightly, use a spoon to remove the flesh.

-Blend the remaining ingredients in a food processor with the eggplant flesh until thoroughly combined.

-Taste for seasoning and make any adjustments.

Nutritional Facts:

Calories: 48 , Fat: 3 g, Carbohydrates: 5 g, Fiber: 3 g

Protein: 2 g

Prep Time: 30 minutes

49. Air Fryer Falafel

Ingredients:

- One (1) can chickpeas, drained and rinsed

- One (1) small onion, minced

- One (2) cloves garlic, minced

- Two (2) tablespoons fresh parsley, chopped

- Two (2) teaspoons ground cumin

- Two (2) teaspoons ground coriander

- One (1) teaspoon baking powder

- Salt and pepper to taste

- Two (2) tablespoons olive oil

Instructions:

-In a food processor, combine all the ingredients (apart from the olive oil) and process until a thick paste develops.

-Create 1-inch balls out of the mixture, then arrange them on a platter.

-Apply a thin layer of olive oil to each falafel ball.

-Falafel balls should be placed in an air fryer basket and cooked at 375°F for 8 to 10 minutes, or until crispy and golden.

-Serve with your favorite dipping sauce, such as tahini.

Nutritional Facts:

Calories: 132 , Fat: 6 g, Carbohydrates: 16 g, Fiber: 5 g

Protein: 5 g

Prep Time: 20 minutes

50. Stuffed Mushrooms

Ingredients:

-Six-Eight large mushrooms, stems removed

- Quarter (1/4) cup walnuts, finely chopped

- Quarter (1/4) cup sun-dried tomatoes, finely chopped

- Two (2) cloves garlic, minced

- Two (2) tablespoons fresh parsley, chopped

- Two (2) tablespoons olive oil

- Salt and pepper to taste

Instructions:

-Set the oven temperature to 400°F and cover baking sheet with parchment paper.

-Sun-dried tomatoes, parsley, garlic, walnuts, olive oil, salt, and pepper should all be combined in a bowl.

-Fill the mixture into each mushroom cap.

-Bake the mushrooms on the baking sheet for 15 to 20 minutes, or until they are just starting to brown.

-Serve warm.

Nutritional Facts:

Calories: 110 , Fat: 8 g, Carbohydrates: 8 g, Fiber: 2 g

Protein: 4 g

Prep Time: 15 minutes

51. Baked Zucchini Fritters

Ingredients:

- Two (2) zucchinis, grated

- Two (2) tablespoons fresh parsley, chopped

- One (1) small onion, minced

- Two (2) cloves garlic, minced

- One (1) teaspoon ground cumin

- Half (1/2) teaspoon smoked paprika

- Half (1/2) cup breadcrumbs

- One (1) tablespoon olive oil

Instructions:

-Set the oven temperature to 375°F and cover baking sheet with parchment paper.

-Place all the ingredients in a bowl and stir to thoroughly incorporate.

-Form mixture into fritters by dividing it into twelve equal parts.

-Put the fritters on the baking sheet and slightly brush with olive oil.

-Bake for 20 to 25 minutes, turning once.

Nutritional Facts:

Calories: 97 , Fat: 4 g, Carbohydrates: 13 g, Fiber: 2 g

Protein: 3 g

Prep Time: 15 minutes

52. Avocado Toast

Ingredients:

- Two (2) slices whole grain bread

- One (1) ripe avocado

- Two (2) tablespoons olive oil

-Salt and pepper to taste

Instructions:

-Bread should be gently toasted till golden.

-Take the avocado flesh out and mash it with a fork.

-Avocado butter and olive oil are spread on toast.

-Add a pinch of salt and pepper.

Nutritional Facts:

Calories: 214 , Fat: 16 g, Carbohydrates: 17 g, Fiber: 5 g

Protein: 4 g

Prep Time: 5 minutes

53. Baked Potato Skins

Ingredients:

- Four (4) large russet potatoes

- Two (2) tablespoons olive oil

- One (1) teaspoon garlic powder

- Half (1/2) teaspoon paprika

-Salt and pepper to taste

-Vegan cheese of your choice (optional)

Instructions:

-Set the oven temperature to 425°F and cover baking sheet with parchment paper.

-Clean potatoes, then slice in half lengthwise.

-Garlic powder, paprika, salt, and pepper should be added after brushing each potato half with olive oil.

-Bake the potatoes for 25 to 30 minutes, or until they are soft, with the sliced side down on the baking sheet.

-Remove the potatoes from the oven and allow them to cool slightly.

-Remove the skin of the potato, leaving approximately a quarter inch of it in the skin, and discard.

-If preferred, add vegan cheese on the top of each potato shell.

-Put the potatoes back in the oven and bake for another 10-15 minutes, or until the cheese is melted and starting to brown.

Nutritional Facts:

Calories: 166 , Fat: 8 g, Carbohydrates: 21 g, Fiber: 3 g

Protein: 2 g

Prep Time: 30 minutes

54. Baked Kale Chips

Ingredients:

- One (1) bunch kale, torn into pieces

- Two (2) tablespoons olive oil

-Salt and pepper to taste

Instructions:

-Set the oven temperature to 350°F and cover baking sheet with parchment paper.

-Add salt and pepper and toss the chopped kale with the olive oil.

-Spread the kale in a single layer on the baking sheet.

-Bake for 10 to 12 minutes, or until crisp and just beginning to brown.

Nutritional Facts:

Calories: 43 , Fat: 3 g, Carbohydrates: 4 g, Fiber: 1 g

Protein: 2 g

Prep Time: 15 minutes

55. Cucumber Tomato Salad

Ingredients:

- Two (2) large cucumbers, diced

- Two (2) large tomatoes, diced

- Two (2) tablespoons olive oil

- Two (2) tablespoons red wine vinegar

- One (1) tablespoon fresh basil, chopped

-Salt and pepper to taste

Instructions:

-In a bowl, add all the ingredients and stir to thoroughly blend.

-Chill for 15 minutes to let flavors mingle.

-Serve chilled.

Nutritional Facts:

Calories: 57 , Fat: 4 g, Carbohydrates: 5 g, Fiber: 2 g

Protein: 1 g

Prep Time: 10 minutes

56. Chili-Lime Edamame

Ingredients:

- One (1) pound frozen edamame

- Two (2) tablespoons olive oil

- One (1) teaspoon chili powder

- One (1) teaspoon garlic powder

- One (1) teaspoon lime juice

-Salt and pepper to taste

Instructions:

-Add edamame to a saucepan of boiling water.

-Edamame should be cooked for 5 minutes or until soft.

-Transfer the drained edamame to a dish.

-Toss the edamame with the olive oil, salt, pepper, lime juice, chili powder, and garlic powder.

-Serve warm.

Nutritional Facts:

Calories: 143 , Fat: 7 g, Carbohydrates: 9 g, Fiber: 5 g

Protein: 10 g

Prep Time: 10 minutes

57. Marinated Tofu

Ingredients:

- One (1) package extra-firm tofu, pressed and cubed

- Quarter (1/4) cup olive oil

- Two (2) cloves garlic, minced

- Two (2) tablespoons fresh oregano, chopped

- Two (2) tablespoons lemon juice

- Two (2) tablespoons red wine vinegar

-Salt and pepper to taste

Instructions:

-In a large bowl, combine all the ingredients and stir until the tofu is thoroughly covered.

-Cover bowl and place in refrigerator to marinate for at least 4 hours. (or overnight).

-Add marinated tofu to a big skillet that is already hot over medium heat.

-Cook for 5-7 minutes, tossing once, or until just lightly browned.

-Serve warm.

Nutritional Facts:

Calories: 183, Fat: 13 g, Carbohydrates: 5 g, Fiber: 1 g

Protein: 11 g

Prep Time: 10 minutes + marinating time

58. Baked Sweet Potato Rounds

Ingredients:

- Two (2) large sweet potatoes, sliced into 1/2 inch rounds

- Two (2) tablespoons olive oil

- One (1) teaspoon garlic powder

-Half (1/2) teaspoon paprika

-Salt and pepper to taste

Instructions:

-Set the oven temperature to 400°F and cover baking sheet with parchment paper.

-Toss the sliced sweet potatoes in the olive oil and seasonings.

-Potato rounds should be arranged in a single layer on the baking sheet.

-Bake for 20 to 25 minutes, turning once.

Nutritional Facts:

Calories: 83 , Fat: 4 g, Carbohydrates: 11 g, Fiber: 2 g

Protein: 1 g

Prep Time: 15 minutes

CHAPTER 5

Plant-Based Meal Planning

Day 1:

Breakfast: Overnight oats with almond milk, banana, and blueberries

Lunch: Quinoa and black bean salad with avocado and tomatoes

Dinner: Vegan chili with brown rice

Day 2:

Breakfast: Smoothie bowl with banana, spinach, almond butter, and chia seeds

Lunch: Lentil and veggie wrap with hummus

Dinner: Baked sweet potato with black beans, spinach, and salsa

Day 3:

Breakfast: Porridge with almond milk, banana, and walnuts

Lunch: Roasted veggies with quinoa and tahini dressing

Dinner: Baked tofu with stir-fried veggies and brown rice

Day 4:

Breakfast: Avocado toast with tomato and basil

Lunch: Chickpea and veggie wrap with hummus

Dinner: Roasted vegetable bowl with quinoa, black beans, and tahini dressing

Day 5:

Breakfast: Oatmeal with almond milk, banana, and almonds

Lunch: Lentil and veggie soup

Dinner: Baked sweet potato with black beans and spinach

Day 6:

Breakfast: Smoothie bowl with banana, spinach, almond butter, and chia seeds

Lunch: Quinoa and black bean salad with avocado and tomatoes

Dinner: Baked tofu with stir-fried veggies and brown rice

Day 7:

Breakfast: Porridge with almond milk, banana, and walnuts

Lunch: Chickpea and veggie wrap with hummus

Dinner: Roasted vegetable bowl with quinoa, black beans, and tahini dressing

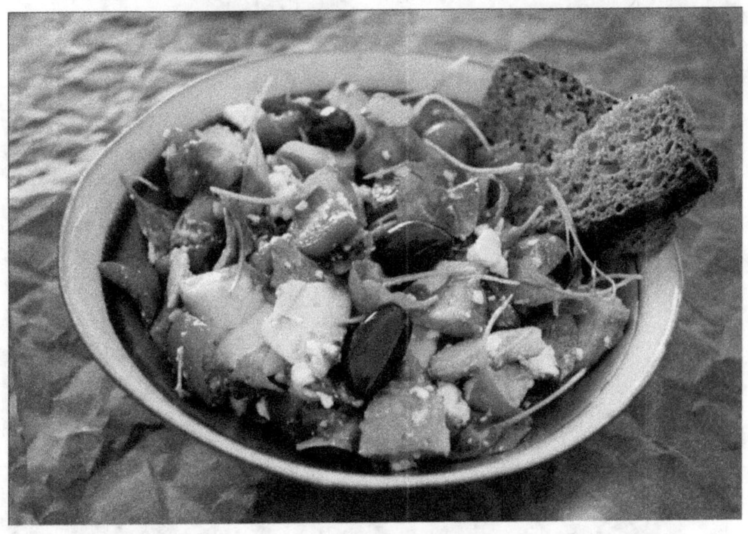

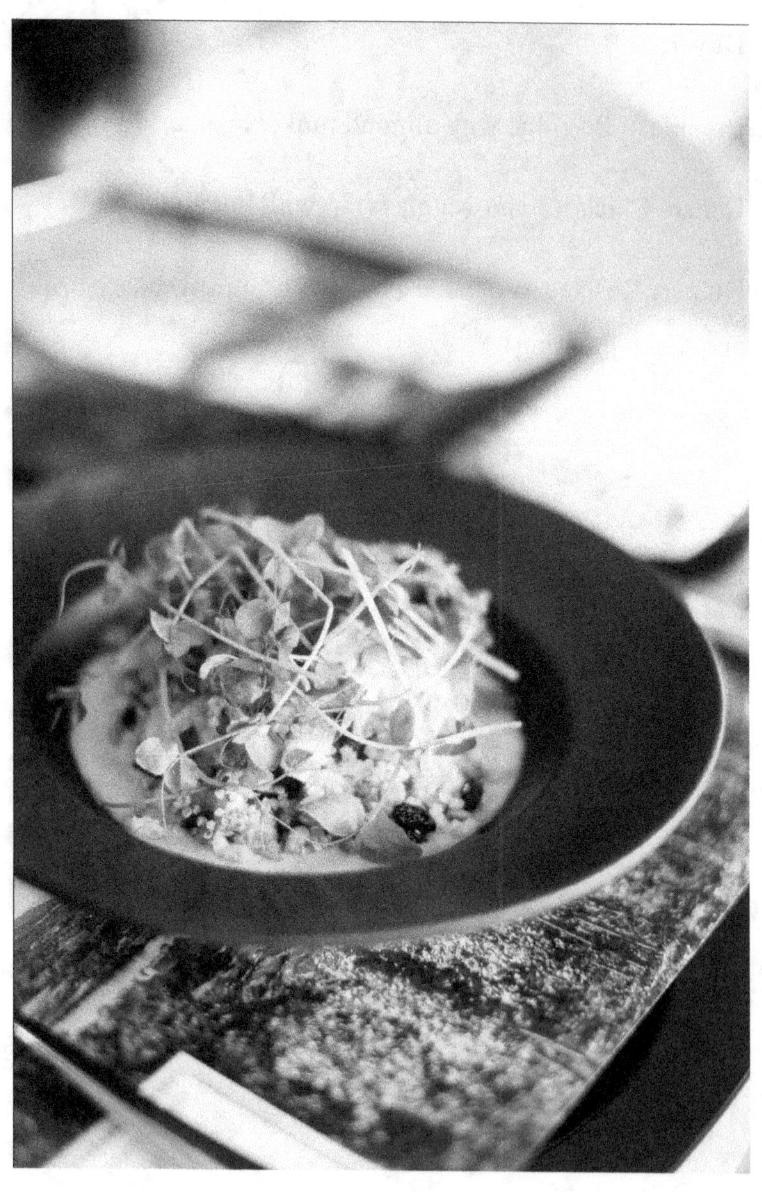

CONCLUSION

The Complete Plant-Based Diet Cookbook is a comprehensive and invaluable resource for anyone looking to transition to a plant-based lifestyle. From simple, delicious breakfasts to creative and flavorful dinners, this cookbook has everything you need to create a plant-based diet that is sure to please everyone. With an emphasis on fresh, whole foods, and an abundance of vegan recipes, this cookbook is a must-have for anyone looking to transition to a plant-based diet.

Anyone wishing to transition to a plant-based diet will find The Complete Plant-Based Diet Cookbook to be a priceless tool. From those who are just starting out to seasoned plant-based veterans, it provides something for everyone with its huge array of dishes. The components are available and reasonably priced, and the recipes are straightforward. The cookbook is also jam-packed with pointers and methods to make your transition as easy and joyful as possible.

In general, The Complete Plant-Based Diet Cookbook is a vital tool for anybody wishing to switch to a more plant-based way of life.

This cookbook will satisfy even the pickiest foodies with its wide variety of delectable and healthy meals.